Herbal Medicines of the Civil War

Published by
Long Creek Herbs
P.O. Box 127
Blue Eye, MO 65611
417-779-5450
www.Longcreekherbs.com

ISBN 1-889791-17-2

Preface

I've been interested in plants that heal for much of my life. As a child, I pestered the oldest adults in my community for their memories of medicinal plants. I read everything I could get my hands on, including unpublished diaries of the 1800s and antique medical texts.

My interest in the Civil War came from discovering an ancestor who served in the Confederate Army. Learning about him, my research revealed he was a prisoner of war. He had been wounded and was treated by both Confederate and Union doctors.

These interests led me to do more research, including attending Civil War encampments and reenactments. Enthusiastic about the materials I found concerning folk healers who were drafted into the War and who became military doctors, I wanted to discuss those issues with reenactors at Civil War events.

Reenactors sometimes get so full of themselves they believe their point of view is the only one that is valid. Many times actors playing Civil War doctors at events have told me, "Boy, you don't know what you're talking about. Military doctors sawed legs and arms off, they didn't waste time using plants!"

My research shows otherwise.

I believe it is misleading to portray a doctor of that time, showing only the dramatic and gory scenes of surgery. Doctors, whether Union surgeons or folk healers, did have to amputate arms and legs when there was no other method of treatment, or when that was the most expedient way to save lives. But there was a respected tradition of healing which used other, less severe methods whenever possible. Plant based medicines were at the heart of those practices.

Introduction

The Civil War was a cauldron of medical experimentation and improvisation. Not that it started out that way, but as the War progressed, elements of diverse American life were thrust together in volatile ways testing the methods and practices used by physicians, folk healers and the old guard military doctors.

This book is a look at the some of the plants used during this time and the formulas made from combining them. Diaries of the period, as well as accounts from doctors, stories in the newspapers and other records, reveal plants played an indispensable part in the healing of the sick and wounded during the Civil War.

When the first shots were fired in April of 1861, the military medical profession was greatly unprepared for the vast numbers of casualties and the wounded they were required to treat. The medical corps was so totally inadequate for dealing with the removal or treatment of large numbers of casualties, wounded men were sometimes left on the battlefield, awaiting treatment, in pouring rain for as long as 48 hours.

However, by the time of the Battle of Gettysburg, in 1863, the efficiency of the medical corps had improved so much that, at the end of each day, not one wounded man was left on the battlefield. This marked the beginning of modern triage in large-scale warfare.

At the beginning of the War, the Union listed only 98 medical officers for the entire Army. Those were predominantly older doctors, near retirement age and without any significant refresher training since the 1840s. The Confederate Army listed only 24 physicians, all of those apparently coming from the tradition of folk healer.

By the end of the Civil War, the Union Army had recorded the services of 11,000 doctors and the Confederates listed 3,000. Additionally some cross-over took place when doctors were captured and forced to continue in service as healers for the other side.

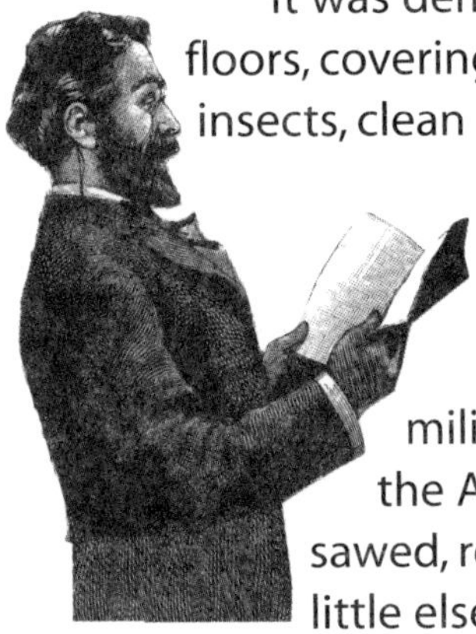

It was demonstrated during the War that cleaner floors, coverings on hospital windows to keep out insects, clean medical instruments, and preventative or early treatment with quinine for malaria, all had positive influences on the healing of patients.

The general assumption by many military reenactors is that all physicians in the Army were surgeons who cut and sawed, removing arms and legs but knowing little else of healing. While military surgeons were required to do those things, a look into the methods of training physicians of that period shows a very different medical discipline. When not simply overwhelmed by the sheer numbers of wounded in major battles, military doctors could do much to treat their patients' wounds, illness and complaints. Unfortunately, treatments were often based on myth rather than science, and healing was accomplished sometimes as much by accident as by design.

Many of the illnesses and injuries of patients during the War were the result of poor, chaotic living conditions rather than actual battle. Historians have estimated that close to 690,000 American soldiers died in the Civil War. Only about 160,000 of those died on the battlefield and another 80,000 died later from wounds. Around 40,000 died from accidents of various kinds, but the largest number by far, about 425,000 men, died from illness and disease. Epidemics of measles were common on both sides. Diarrhea and dysentery were rampant. Diarrhea, dysentery, typhoid, malaria and pneumonia killed more soldiers on both sides than gunfire.

Why? Primarily because of profound unsanitary living conditions. Germs and bacteria were not known about and the modern notions of hygiene, diet and sanitation (even simple sanitation) by doctors, were still years away.

Some battles were never fought because of the large

numbers of sick soldiers on both sides. Soldiers filled their canteens from the same streams where they bathed, where animals stood and relieved themselves.

There were various treatments for diarrhea and dysentery. Some worked marginally while others were totally useless. What would have solved the problems would have been unspoiled food and clean water. Even when a doctor offered a remedy for these ailments, something like charcoal and wild lettuce *(Latuca canadensis)* or syrup of green persimmon, soldiers became sick again from drinking the same water and eating the same spoiled food.

Misconceptions abounded as to the causes of these diseases, including "bad air," eating unsalted beef and, "The Humors" (or vapors), arising from swamps.

Infection was expected, even welcomed, in the treatment of wounds and thought to be a necessary aspect of healing. A doctor might operate on patients throughout the day in the battlefield hospital, never cleaning his medical instruments with the exception of wiping them off on his coattails or on the shirts of patients.

It soon became apparent, however, that doctors who washed their instruments in hot water, who regularly replaced sawdust on hospital floors, and who covered hospital windows with cloth to keep out insects, demonstrated higher rates of successful healing than the doctors who didn't do those things. But the science of medicine was still in its infancy.

The American Medical Association had been formed in 1847, with the specific purpose of elevating the doctor from the category of a tradesman to that of a professional, and to establish standards for training. School terms were regulated by the AMA to two 6 month terms, to be followed by proof of internship. By 1850 this system was producing licensed doctors, although no system of enforcement existed. The general practice continued to be learning by apprenticeship until after the Civil War.

The average doctor in the Civil War was from a rural background and had been apprenticed to another doctor to learn his trade. He relied upon his skills with herbs and plants, often digging from the wild, a good portion of his medicines.

Opium, from poppies, and whiskey were the common pain killers. These were generally combined with cayenne. (Cayenne, when added to a medicine, causes the medicine to be absorbed into the body faster. The use of cayenne in medicine is generally thought to have arrived from the Southwest with the opening of the Santa Fe Trail.)

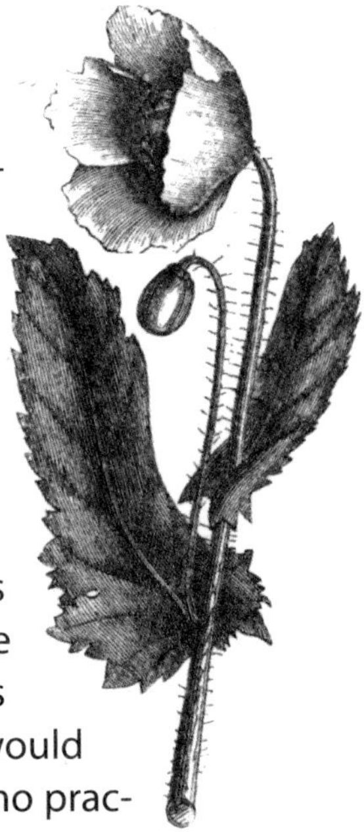

Some popular and commonly accepted medicines of the time, such as compounds of mercury, nitric acid, turpentine and creosote, were often lethal to the body. Each of these were usually combined with doses of whiskey or brandy and given as medicines and generally did more harm than good.

There were a few medical schools, each of those having two or three professors who initially established the school as a means of making a personal profit. In the beginning these so-called medical schools had no testing or licensing and a doctor would be graduated in a year's time having had no practical, hands-on experience with treating patients. The method of teaching was to have students sit in a lecture hall and listen to lectures without ever having picked up a medical instrument, mixed medicines or seen a patient!

There was virtually no official training for nurses before the War, with the exception of one nursing school near Philadelphia, established in 1850. By and large, nursing care not provided by families was performed either by slaves in the South or by religious orders in the North.

The common method for training doctors up to this time was by apprenticeship. The apprentice generally paid, on average, about $100 a year for a two year apprenticeship with a practicing physician. During that time the apprentice learned how to dig roots, grind herbs, mix medical formulas, prepare salves and tinctures. Additionally the apprentice was responsible for chopping wood, cleaning house, caring for horses and any other duties the doctor required. He was expected to learn formulas for medicines, identify plants and learn about diseases.

The big advantage of the apprenticeship method was in allowing the physician in training to accompany the doctor on house calls and help in the actual treatment of patients. He learned about delivering babies, treating wounds, applying medicines, setting broken bones. An apprentice thereby gained a skill level often exceeding those early medical school trained physicians.

With this system of apprenticeship there was a certain degree of continuity, and even a common man could become a doctor. And it was men, who became doctors. Women were almost completely denied access to the profession of medicine. The lone recorded exception was Dr. Elizabeth Blackwell, who was graduated from Geneva Medical College in 1849.

"Urging upon the medical officers the necessity for collecting the indigenous botanical remedies of the South and employing them liberally in the treatment of the sick. The indigenous, the cranes-bill, the marsh rosemeary (sic) blackberry, sweet gum and others should be made available...

The above quote is from the Surgeon-General's Office in Richmond, Virginia. He was writing to instruct the field commanders to order their physicians to call upon their skills of herbs and plants. The efficacy of plant based medicine was already in common practice, as I have indicated, and the potential for new discoveries had been dramatically demonstrated.

The mixing of cultures, which accelerated throughout the 1800s, included influences from the Spanish, the French, the British and Native Americans. From the 1820s to 1847, the Santa Fe Trail had a powerful influence on medicines of later periods, especially those of the Civil War.

Commerce with the East, via St. Louis, and with the Southwest, saw the addition of new medicines traveling both ways along the Trail. The revolutionary "new" treatment for malaria, first showcased in Philadelphia, soon became standard on trails west.

Dr. John Sappington, who studied in Philadelphia where quinine was first introduced, began manufacturing "Sappington's Little Pills" in Arrow Rock, Missouri in the 1830s. This form of quinine, derived from a South American tree, is credited with having made travel along both the Santa Fe and Oregon Trails far less life threatening.

But at the beginning of the Civil War, it was still a common practice for military doctors to treat malaria by bleeding and purging the patient before using the anti-malaria medicine, quinine. Even though it was standard practice for medical doctors outside the military to use quinine as the first line of treatment for the previous twenty years (without the use of purging and bleeding), the military was slow to accept this more progressive treatment.

A folk healer who found himself working as a physician in the military during the War, often had previous exposure to regional folk practices and even some limited Native American methods. While the military surgeon might have been tempted to simply amputate an arm that was hit with a bullet which broke bones, the folk healer, using older traditions, often did not. Instead, he would treat the wound, usually with something to stop the bleeding such as yarrow *(Achillea milefolium)*. Yarrow had a reputation for blood stopping on the battlefield that dates from early Roman and Greek times.

He would then set the bone by an Indian method that had proven useful. A small animal, usually a raccoon or 'possum, would be killed and skinned. A poultice of plants would be administered to the wound, then the fresh hide of the animal would be applied, fur side out, and tied in place.

The skin would slowly shrink, tightening around the wound and broken bone. The bone would be slowly pulled back into place and the animal hide would be left in place for about two weeks, forming a cast for the wound. There was no need to amputate the arm when it could be saved! Many healers during that time knew this method and would not remove an arm that could be salvaged.

Any men skilled in the healing arts, particularly those who could adapt their methods to field conditions, were likely to be pressed into service for the daily, emergency, or aftercare of soldiers on both sides throughout the Civil War. At a time when medical licensing was just beginning, a wealth of plant based healing practices from various cultures were employed and found useful.

I hope the information contained in this book might cause those who study the Civil War period to recognize and look further for examples of plant based treatments and healing.

A Time Line of Certain Advances in Modern Medicine

- 1831 Chloroform introduced
- 1832 Quinine introduced
- 1842 Ether first used, but not published until 1849, and not generally used until near the end of the Civil War
- 1845 Band aids invented, although not generally used until after the War
- 1853 Hypodermic needle introduced
- 1854 The first local anesthetic administered with the hypodermic needle

The Plants

It is impossible to list all of the medicinal plants used during the time of the Civil War, simply because there were so many. Materia Medica and Pharmacopeia of the time list thousands, including both imported as well as indigenous medicinal plants. Many are still used today, although often not in the same ways as in the past. Here is a listing of some of the plants used by physicians of the time.

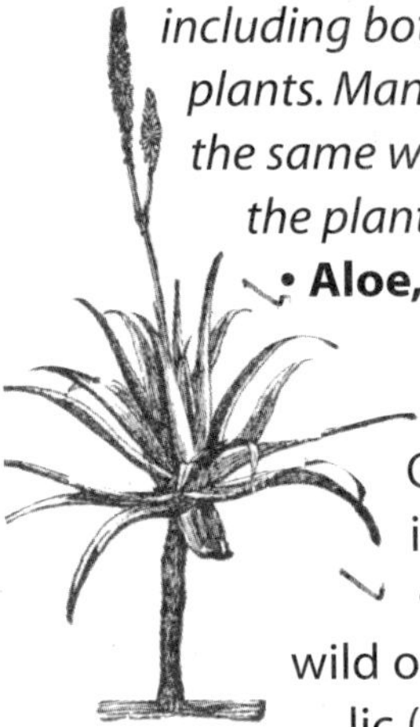

Aloe perryi
also known as
"Cape Aloe"

• **Aloe,** both imported varieties as well as our native *Aloe vera* were used, generally as a purgative and sometimes poultice. Often listed as "Cape Aloes" in older medical texts.

• **Allium** - Onion/Garlic. Both domestic and wild onions (*A. tricoccum* & related sp.) and garlic (*A. sativum*) were used for treating wounds, skin infections and insect stings. Both have antibacterial properties and were used up until World War I, medicinally.

• **Alumroot** *(Heuchera americana)* - Used similarly to alum as a styptic and astringent for wounds, piles, gargle for sore throat, sores, wounds, abrasions as well as treating diarrhea and dystentery. *See also page 28.*

• **Anthemidis** - Chamomile *(Anthemis nobilis);* used as a stimulant and antispasmodic in large does and as a simple tonic, sleep inducer and relaxer in smaller doses.

• **Asafetida** *(Ferula assafoetida)* - Used as an amulet, worn on a string around the neck as it was believed to ward off illness. Used as a seasoning

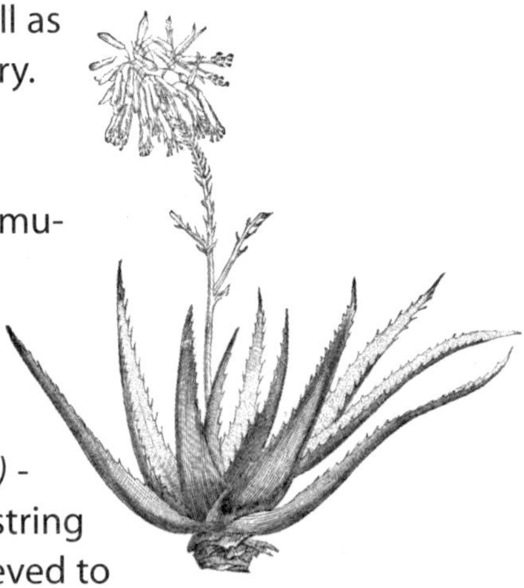

Aloe vera

herb in small amounts in many Asian and Indian cultures and also the "secret" ingredient in Worchestshire sauce.

• **Bee-Balm** (*Monarda fistulosa* & related sp.) - as a tea for colic, upset stomach, to induce sweating, poulticed leaves for headaches.

• **Blackberry** *(Rubus villosus)*) & **Black Raspberry** *(Rubus occidentalis)* used as astringent, tonic tea for diarrhea, dystentery, stomach pain, gonorrhea, "female tonic," leaf wash for sores.

• **Bloodroot** *(Sanguinaria canadensis)* - Historically used in cough medicines, sedative, appetite stimulant and root juice applied to warts and as a dye plant.

• **Blue Vervain** *(Verbena hastata)* - American Indians used this plant in a tonic for women, also used historically for coughs, intestinal problems, dysentery, stomach cramps. Root preferred over leaves but both were used.

• **Boneset/Thoroughwort** *(Eupatorium perfoliatum)* - Leaf tea used to induce sweating, to treat flu; also used for pleurisy, pneumonia, gout, and as antispasmodic; leaves poulticed on tumors. Large doses emetic.

• **Burdock** *(Arctium lappa & A. minus)* - Diaphoretic, diuretic, alterative, used for treating rheumatism, gout, psoriasis, acne, burns, wounds, swellings.

• **Calendula** *(Calendula officinalis)* - Often listed as Pot Marigold, although it is not in the marigold family. Anti-inflammatory, eyewash, poultice on skin conditions, used in salves for skin ailments. In the book, ***Dictionary of Terms Used in Medicine*** by Richard Hoblyn, 1846...*"Marygold; a well-known garden plant, formerly much used in medicine and thought to be antispasmodic, sudorific, deobstruent and emmenagogue. It is now rarely employed."*

• **Canadian Snakeroot** - See Ginger, wild. There are many plants listed colloquilly as "snakeroot" and without the Latin name, can often be confusing. Canadian Snakeroot was a common name for the native *Asarum canadense*.

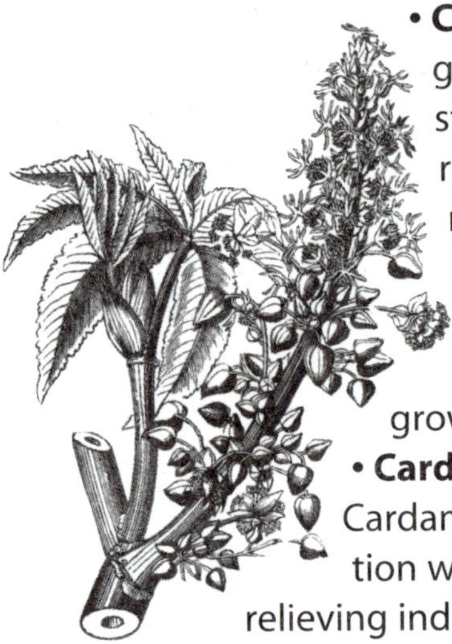

Castor Bean
(Ricinus communis)
Source of castor oil

• **Canna** *(Canna edulis)* - Rhiizomes ground under water, kneading, straining then allowing to evaporate. The resulting powder used as nutritive food for urinary and bowel affections in invalids, infants and in convalescense. Not broadly available but increasingly grown in the Southern states.

• **Cardamom** seed, often listed as Cardamomi; generally used in combination with other medications and for relieving indigestion.

• **Castor bean** *(Ricinus communis)* Oil used as laxative and purgative in food poisoning; used externally for ringworm, sores and hair wash for dandruff. Note: seeds are a deadly poison.

• **Catnip** *(Nepeta cataria)* - Folk remedy for bronchitis, colds, diarrhea, fevers, headaches, inducing sleep, promoting sweating. Used as well as antispasmodic and in treating hysteria and colic. Also used in Europe as a dream or comfort pillow, especially with very young babies to help them sleep through the night.

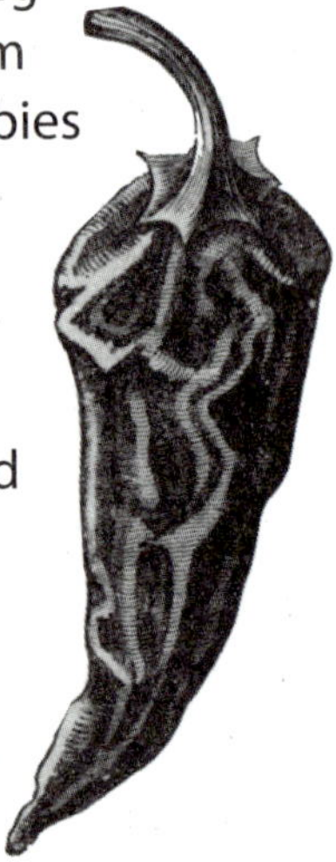

• **Cayenne pepper** - *Pulveris capsicum*; powdered red pepper. Used as a topical rubefacient (to raise blisters or cause reddening of the skin) and given orally with other medications to speed absorption into the bloodstream. Sometimes spelled colloquially as "cyan" and "cian" pepper, and listed as "capsicum."

• **Chamomile** *(Chamomilla recutita*, also listed as *Matricaria chamomilla)*; also known as wild or German chamomile; dried flowers used as relaxing tea for sleep aid, for upset stomach, also used in treating diarrhea, gout, fevers, flu and other ailments.

• **Chicory** *(Cichorium intybus)* - Used in treatment for jaundice, as a diuretic, laxative, to lower blood sugar, for liver and gall bladder ailments. Also combined (roasted roots) with dried roots of dandelion as coffee substitute.

• **Colt's Foot** *(Tussilago farfara)* - Leaf and flower traditionally used for sore throats, coughs, asthma, bronchitis.

• **Columbine** *(Aquilegia canadensis)* - Astringent, diuretic; Native Americans used crushed seeds for headaches. Also used in treating fevers and seeds ground and mixed with lard to control head lice.

• **Cohosh, Black** *(Cimicifuga racemosa)* - Tincture used for bronchitis, fevers, snakebites, menstrual irregularities. *See Rattle Root.*

• **Cohosh, Blue** *(Caulophyllum thalictroides)* - Root tea used extensively by Native Americans as aid in labor, to treat profuse menstruation, cramping, urinary tract infections, inflammation of the uterus. This was one of the important ingredients in the Lydia Pinkham's compound for women, popular after the Civil War.

• **Colocynth** *(Citrullus colocynthis)* - Like many medicines of the time, this is a cathartic; also listed as liver stimulant, diuretic. In very small doses used as stomachic; in large doses a strong emetic, irritant, poison. Used by early Greeks and Arabians. Very harsh and seldom used by itself.

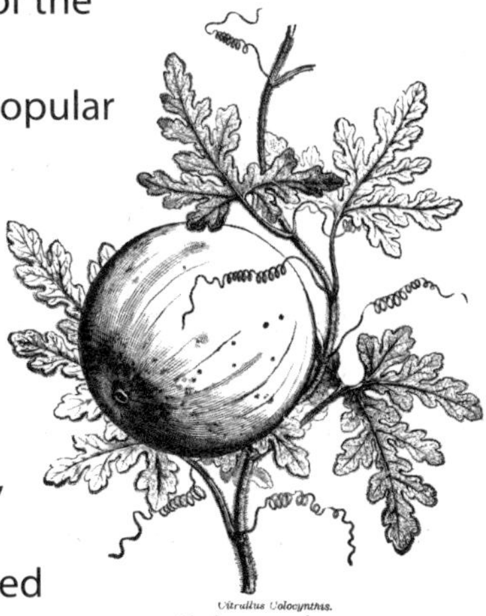

Colocynth

• **Colombo** - A tropical vine from eastern Africa. In small doses used to augment liver secretion, in larger doses produces diarrhea, vomiting and tremors.

• **Compass-Plant** *(Silphium laciniatum)* and Prairie Dock *(Silphium terebinthinaceum)* - Both used in folk medicine for general tonic, emetic, coughs; root tea used in treatment of gonorrhea and asthma.

• **Coneflower** *(Echinacea sp.)* - Listed in some old sources as "snakeroot" (many plants are listed under that name); used in infections, chronic inflammations, for treatments on wounds, canker sores, spider bites and many other uses.

• **Cotton** *(Gossypium herbaceum)* - Used as absorbent in bandages; macerated with solvents to make collodium, a liquid, protective bandage. Roots employed as abortifacient by Southern slave women.

• **Culver's-Root** *(Veronicastrum virginicum)* - Used as strong laxative, to induce sweating, induce vomiting. Dried root part used.

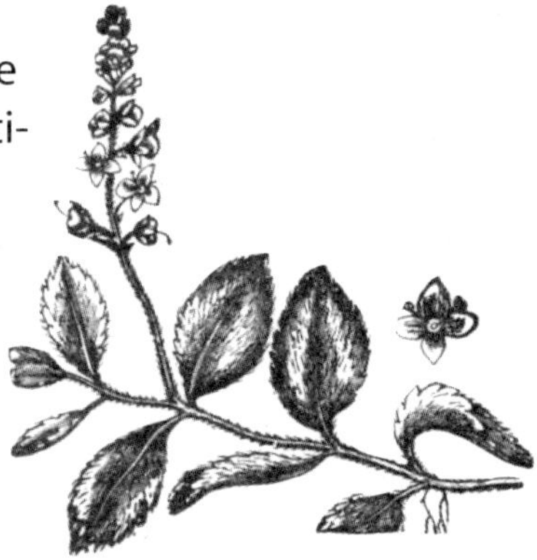
Culver's-Root
(Veronicastrum virginicum)

• **Crocus, autumn** *(Crocus autumnale*, earlier listing as *Colchicum autumnale)* - In small amounts is alterative, cathartic, emetic, sedative and diuretic, used in treatment of gout for centuries. Highly poisonous and used only with caution. Not to be confused with *Crocus sativum*, the saffron crocus, which also blooms in the fall but is not poisonous.

• **Dandelion** *(Taraxacum officinale)* - Tea of fresh root traditionally used for gall bladder, liver, kidney and bladder problems; also as a tonic for poor digestion; dried leaf used as a laxative.

• **Elcampane** *(Inula helenium)* - Non-indigenous species; root tea used to treat pneumonia,whooping cough, bronchitis, stomach problems and worm expellant.

• **Elderberry** *(Sambucus canadensis)* - Bark tea used as diuretic, laxative; leaves poulticed on sores, cuts and to stop bleeding. Both leaves & bark used in healing salves. Decoction of leaves/bark used as wash for eczema, skin conditions.

• **Epazote, Wormseed** *(Chenopodium ambrosioides)* - Purgative to expel worms, condiment in Mexican bean dishes.

• **Fennel** *(Foeniculum vulgare)* - Teas used to relieve gas, colic in infants, and stimulating milk flow.

• **Feverfew** *(Chrysanthemum parthenium)* - Escaped from cultivation early in 1800s. Proven effective (1-4 fresh leaves chewed per day) for treating some kinds of migraine headaches; is also antiseptic. Rarely causes allergic dermatitis and mouth sores in some people.

• **Flaxseed** - Often listed in medical texts as *Pulveris Lini;* used in inflammation of the gastrointestinal tract. Flaxseed was also ground, moistened with boiling water and applied as poultice for wounds.

• **Foxglove** *(Digitalis purpurea)* - Used in folk medicine (as well as in modern times) to treat heart problems. Can be lethally toxic if used as self medication. Other names for this plant include Dead Men's Bells, Dog's Finger, Fairy Gloves, Thimbles and Lion's Mouth.

• **Gentian** *(Gentiana quinquefolia)* - Often listed as Ague-Weed, bitter-root or genciana. Considered the best bitters for encouraging digestion and appetite, as late as 1916 in ***The National Standard Dispensatory***.

• **Ginger**, imported *(Zingiber sp.)* - The genus includes 80 some species, all from tropical to semi-tropical regions. Ginger was imported for medicine in the treatment of stomach problems, indigestion, motion sickness.

• **Ginger**, wild *(Asarum canadense)* - American Indians and early folk healers used the root tea for indigestion, coughs, "female ailments," to relieve gas, promote sweat, and for fevers, colds and sore throats. Sometimes listed as "Canadian snakeroot" in old herbals. Candied wild ginger roots were a sweet treat during the Holidays in some regions.

• **Ginseng** *(Panax quinquefolius)* - Tonic, used to "strengthen the stomach and memory," according to ***The Indian Physician,*** 1828.

• **Goldenseal** *(Hydrastis canadensis)* - Tea, from the root, used to treat mouth, throat, digestive system, uterus, folk remedy for eye infections; believed to restore and strengthen appetite.

• **Holly** *(Ilex sp.)* - Several hollies were used during this time. *Ilex vomitoria*, for example, gets its name from the emetic effect. Porcher, in ***Resources of the Southern Fields & Forests***, 1863 says, "I would particularly recommend the holly root as an article for the relief of colds and coughs. It increases appetite and is a tonic...leaves as a diaphoretic, employed in catarrh, pleurisy, smallpox, etc."

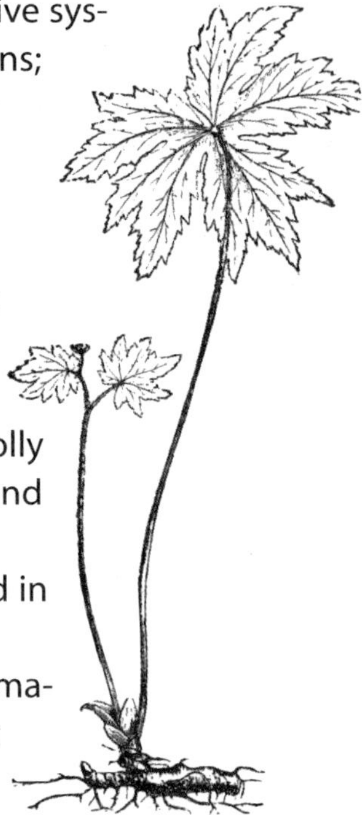

Goldenseal
(Hydrastis canadensis)

• **Hollyhock** *(Althea officinalis)* - In pharmacy the powdered root is very absorbent and used to harden pills. Root and leaves are demulcent, emollient, protective, used in inflammations of pulmonary, digestive and urinary organs, for vaginal and rectal irritation. *Malva sylvestris* also used the same way, both in syrups and as poultice (as recent as ***Materia Medica***, 1927).

• **Hops** *(Humulus lupulus)* - Tea from fruits used as sedative and antispasmodic; also used to treat boils, fevers, cramps, coughs and externally for bruises. Introduced for growing commercially in New York in 1629 and in Virginia in 1648.

• **Horehound** *(Marrubium vulgare)* - Common treatment for coughs, bronchitis, sore throat, stomach and gall bladder problems; fresh leaves poulticed on wounds and cuts.

• **Horseradish** *(Amoracia rusticana)* - ***Hoblyn's***, 1855, lists Horseradish, giving the reference to "horse" to mean, "great, strong." Condiment and occasional use as poultice and plaster.

• **Hyssop** *(Hyssopus officinalis)* - Used since Biblical times as cathartic and wound herb; more recently as stimulant, for rheumatism, bruises, sore throat.

• **Indian Physic** *(Gillenia stipulacea & trifoliata)* - Used as substitute for Ipecac; emetic.

• **Ipecac**, wild *(Euphorbia ipecacuanhae)* - Native plant to the U.S., used as extremely strong laxative, in the purging and bleeding treatments of the early 1800s. This is not the same plant as the imported Ipecac *(Cephaelis ipecacuanha)* but used similarly.

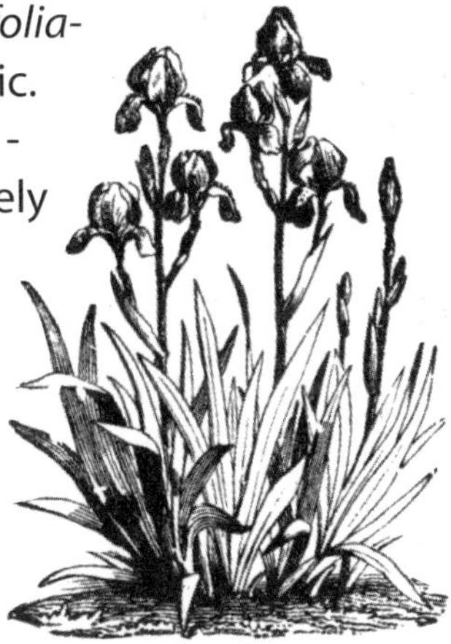
Blue Flag

• **Iris, Blue Flag** *(Iris versicolor)* - Dried rhizome part used; emetic, diuretic, used also in malarial jaundice, remittent fever, dropsy; is very nauseating and prostrating; liver stimulant similar to *Podophyllum*, more pungent than *Euonymous*. Native plant used by Indians as poultice (root) on swellings, bruises, sores; tea as a strong laxative.

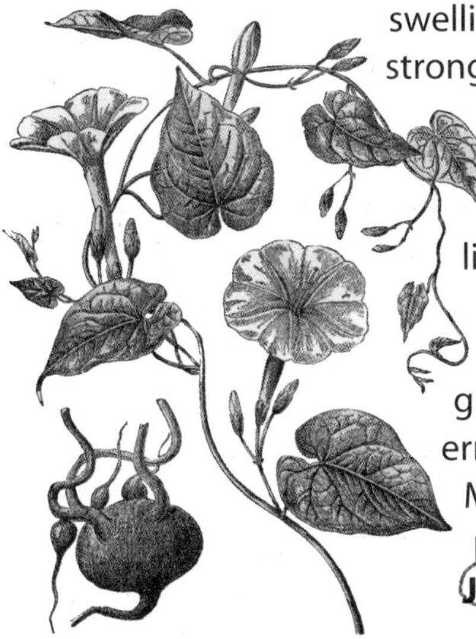
Jalap *(Exogonium jalapa)*

• **Jalap** - Often listed as *Pulveris Jalap* or pulverized Jalap in many older texts; botanically listed as late as 1927 as *Exogonium jalapa*. It is the dried tuberous root of a morning-glory-like vine found on the eastern slopes of the mountains of Mexico. Used primarily as a purgative.

Jewelweed *(Impatiens capensis)* - Crushed leaves poulticed on recent poison ivy, juicy stems crushed and applied to rashes, poison ivy, insect bites, eczema.

• **Larkspur** *(Delphinium sp.)* - Several native larkspurs were used for controlling body and head lice, itch-mites, and for rheumatism and neuralgia; also used as a wound herb. Rarely used internally.

• **Lavender** *(Lavendula sp.)* - Used as flavoring in medicines as well as used in stomach and headache treatments; often combined with other herbs to make antiseptic washes, treatments for rashes and skin problems.

• **Lemon Balm** *(Melissa officinalis)* - The physician, Paracelsus (1493-1541) chose lemon balm for his famous elixir that was purported to regenerate the strength of man. In Civil War times it was added as flavoring and sometimes as fragrant ingredient in teas and decoctions. Also an ingredient in several historically famous colognes.

• **Licorice** *(Glycyrrhiza glabra)* - Often listed as Extract of Glycyrrhiza; used in conjunction with flax seed for treating coughs, sore throat, laryngitis. Also widely used as a flavoring in other medicines.

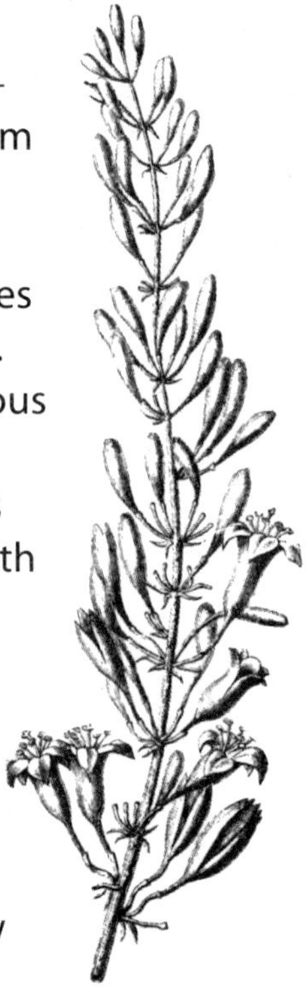
Lavandula officinalis

• **Life Everlasting** - The problem with common names, especially when looking back a century or more, is that several plants may have gone by the same name. What we know today by the common name of life everlasting is a variety of *Sedum*. But old medical texts list several plants by that name, including *Gnaphalium obtusifolium*, also known as sweet everlasting and rabbit tobacco. That plant was used (leaves and flowers, chewed) for sore throats, pneumonia, as well as in teas for colds, fevers, upset stomach, etc. Fresh juice considered as an aphrodisiac.

• **Lobelia, Indian Tobacco** *(Lobelia inflata)* - Also called, "Pukeweed" because of its use to induce vomiting. Also used as sedative, but strongly emetic.
• **Lobelia, Great** *(Lobelia siphilitica)* - Root tea once used to treat syphillis, leaf tea for colds, stomach problems, worms, nosebleeds, gargle for coughs and sore throat.
• **Magnolia, Cucumber** *(Magnolia acuminata)* - Bark tea used as substitute for Cinchona, which was the source of quinine for treating malaria. Also used for indigestion, worms, toothaches, stomach problems.
• **Magnolia, Sweetbay** *(Magnolia virginiana)* - Used in treating colds, warming the blood in spring and other uses similar to Cucumber Magnolia for intermittent fever (malaria) and catarrah. Given as tincture, decoction or infusion.
• **Marshmallow** *(Althea officianalis)* - Used for inflammations of pulmonary, digestive and urinary organs as well as for skin eruptions, herpes, and for vaginal and rectal irritation. Hollyhock *(Althea rosea)* and *Malva sylvestris*, a related garden plant, also used similarly. Part used: root, dried or fresh.
• **Marsh Rosemary** *(Statice limonium var. caroliniana)* - Root in dysentery, for mouth sores, hemorrhages, also in infusion , tincture and decoction. Listed as late as 1927 in ***Materia Medica***.
• **Mayapple** *(Podophyllum peltatum)* - Also called American Mandrake, Duck's Foot, Umbrella Plant. Historically used as strong purgative, internal cleanser, vermifuge. Resin used to treat warts, although resin can cause skin reactions.
• **Mistletoe** *(Phoradendron serotinum)* - Used for headaches, epilepsy (called "fits" in early days), debility, paralysis and as oral contraceptive.
• **Monarda** *(Monarda fistulosa)* - Also known as bergamot, beebalm, Oswego tea. There are many cultivated varieties of this plant but the native *M. fistulosa* and *M. didyma* are the ones most often connected to folk medicines for expelling worms, gas, for stomachaches, nosebleeds, insomnia, poulticed leaves for headaches and for inducing sweating.

• **Mugwort** *(Artemisia vulgaris)* - Leaf tea used as diuretic, to induce sweating, regulates menstrual irregularity and as a nerve tonic; also used in small amounts in pillows to aid in sleeping.

• **Mullein** *(Verbascum thapsus)* - Leaf and flower used as expectorant and antispasmodic; leaves poulticed for tumors, ulcers, piles; stalk used for cramps, fevers and migraines.

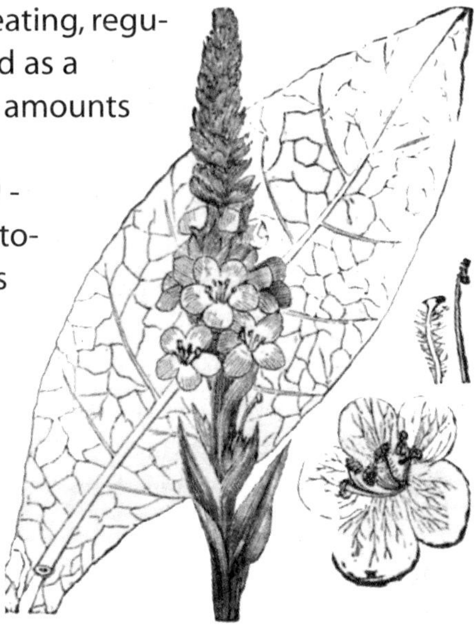

Mullein
(Verbascum thapsus)

• **Mustard seed** - specifically black mustard, used as a laxative, to promote digestion and in plasters for rheumatism, arthritis and headache.

• **New England Aster** *(Aster novae-angliae)* - Root tea used for diarrhea, fevers.

• **New Jersey Tea** *(Ceanothus americanus)* - American Indians used tea from the root for colds, fevers, snakebites, stomach problems, laxative, tonic. Tea of leaves was a popular beverage, being a good substitute for black tea, which was in short supply in the South during the War Between the States. *See also p. 28.*

• **Olive Oil** *(Olea europea)* - Used for a wide variety of purposes, made from the berry of the olive tree. It was, and still is, used for treating gall-stones and as a carrying agent in salves, soaps. Some mystique existed because it was an imported, and therefore, higher quality or mysterious, material. Some physicians of the time (see references in ***"It Will Do No Harm to Try It,"*** by this author) to olive oil by itself being used for rheumatism, arthritis, wounds, etc.

• **Oxalis, Wood Sorrel** *(Oxalis acetosella and O. violacca)* - Porcher said, "The plant is a very agreeable and wholesome salad and possesses refrigerant, antiscorbutic and antiseptic properties...the expressed juice of the plant, much diluted with water, may be used as a good refrigerant drink in fevers....making a refreshing and wholesome conserve with fine sugar; its flavor resembles green tea."

• **Pawpaw** *(Asimina triloba)* - Green fruit is laxative; leaves are insecticidal, also applied to old wounds and absesses. Powdered seeds were common treatment for head lice due to the insecticidal properties. Sometimes listed as custard apple. A soldier could smell the the edible fruit in the woods when ripe.

• **Pennyroyal, American** *(Hedoma pulegioides)* - Tea, from leaves, used to treat colds, coughs, fevers, headaches, to promote sweating and as insect repellent. Calamint *(Satureja arkansana)* also used similarly and has very similar fragrance and taste. Both plants were used by soldiers, simply rubbed onto the skin, to deter ticks, chiggers and mosquitoes. Also packed into bedding and clothing for detering insects.

• **Peppermint** *(Mentha piperita)* - Used as an appetite stimulant, for upset stomach, vomiting and other stomach and digestive problems. Used to flavor drinks and candies as well as being used medicinally.

• **Persimmon** *(Diospyros virginiana)* - Inner bark tea gargled for sore throat; bark tea used as folk remedy for stomachache, diarrhea, dysentery; bark tea also as wash or poultice for cancers, warts. Green fruit boiled down with molasses, sugar or honey to make a thick syrup. Civil War soldiers from the south often carried green persimmon syrup with them as treatment for diarrhea and related stomach and intestinal problems.

• **Peruvian Bark** *(Chinchona succirubra)* - Peruvian bark was used by native peoples in South America for centuries in treating and preventing malaria. However, two Catholic priests "discovered" the herb and brought it to Europe and America. Source of Quinine, which was turned into pills by Dr. John Sappington, in Missouri, in the 1830s and which made travel on the Trails west, possible. At the beginning of the War, most military doctors still practiced blood letting and purging before treating the patient with malaria, with doses of quinine. But well into the War, the medical profession accepted the standards set by Sappington and others and ceased the blood letting and purging as part of the treatment, using only quinine as treatment.

• **Pilewort** *(Erechtities hieracifolia)* - Tea from any part of the plant used internally as astringent; externally for sciatica. Used in diarrhea and related ailments.

• **Pink root** *(Spigelia marilandica)* - Indians and settlers, including soldiers, used root tea as an expellent for intestinal parasites in children and adults.

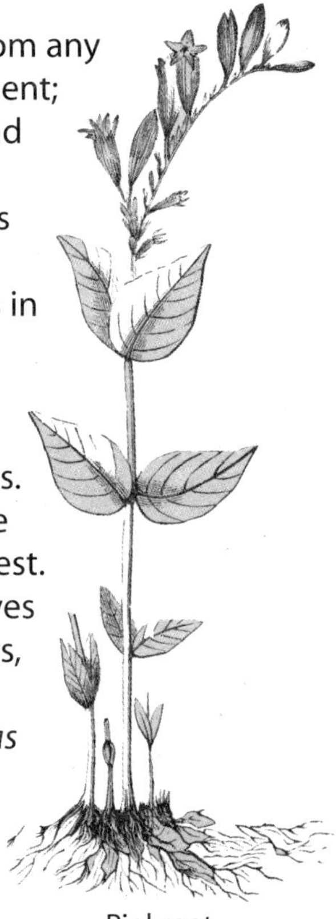

Pinkroot
(Spigelia marilandica)

• **Plantain,** Common *(Plantago major)* & Narrow-Leaf *(P. lanceolata)* - Not a native U.S. plant, but spread by very early settlers. Indians called the plant, "footprints of the white man" as it sprung up along trails West. Used for treating diarrhea, dysentery, leaves used to treat blisters, wounds, sores, ulcers, swelling, insect stings.

• **Pleurisy-root, Butterfly Weed** *(Asclepias tuberosa)* - Root tea traditionally used to treat inflammations of the lungs (pleurisy) as well as asthma and bronchitis. Roots used in poultice for swellings, bruises.

• **Poke Weed** *(Phytolacca americana)* - Skin diseases, scabies, eczema, laxative, emetic. A folk remedy for arthritis was made from berries, steeped in alcohol. Many sources consider the root and berries to be poisonous, although they were used both internally and externally, with care, during the War.

• **Poppy** *(Papaver somniferum)* - The most important pain reliever for many centuries. Mentioned by Homer as an important medicine. Opium and morphine were extracted from the poppy resin and every doctor carried it in either powder or tincture form.

• **Poppy, Prickly** *(Argemone albiflora)* - Emetic, purgative; infusion used for skin ailments, colds, wounds.

• **Prickly Pear Cactus** *(Opuntia humifsa)* - Peeled pads used as poultices on wounds and rheumatism, juice of the fruits to treat warts, tea made from the pads for lung ailments; pads cooked and eaten as vegetable, fruits dried and eaten as a date like sweet confectionary. Larger needles used to remove splinters in hands.

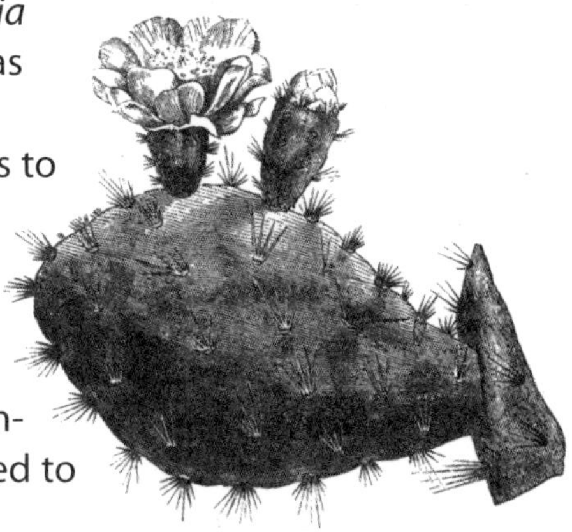

Prickly Pear Cactus
(Opuntia humifsa)

• **Raspberry** *(Rubus sp.)* - Syrups, brandies and tinctures of berries used in bowel problems; root tea for diarrhea, dysentery, stomach pain, back-pain, "female tonic;" leaf tea used as a wash for sores, ulcers, boils. Leaves of both black and red raspberry used for pleasant tea.

• **Rose** *(Rosa sp.)* - Rose hips used for tea; oil from flowers used as fragarnce in the sickroom to mask other odors.

• **Rosemary** *(Rosmarinus officinalis)* - Used for colic, nervous disorders, menstrural problems; externally in rheumatism, sprains, bruises. Mainly used in liniments, lotions, ointments and perfumery.

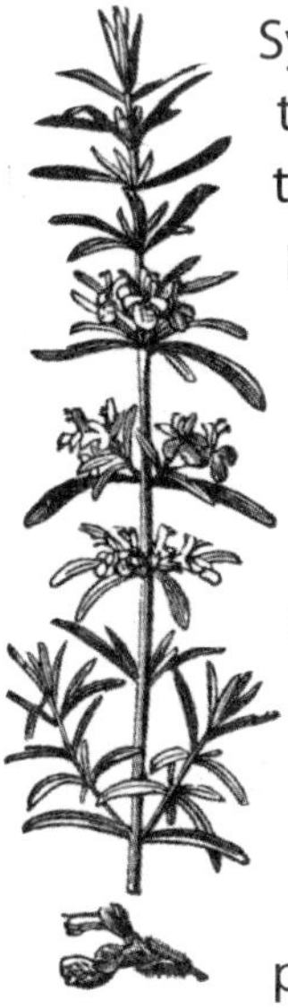

Rosemary

• **Rue** *(Ruta graveolens)* - Stimulating tea in small doses, also used in treating nervous conditions. Can cause convulsions, vomiting and abdominal pain if misused.

• **Rattle Root** *(Cimicifuga racemosa)* - Also listed variously as Rattleroot, Ratil root, Rattleweed, Squawroot and Black Cohosh. Tincture used for nervous disorders, rheumatism, snakebite, menstrual irregularities, childbirth. Lydia Pinkham used this plant in her famous Lydia Pinkham's Compound for Women of the 1870s and beyond. *See also Cohosh, Black, page 13.*

• **Rhubarb** *(Rheum officinale)* - This is not the garden rhubarb, but rather, the Chinese medicinal plant. Generally given as an extract or a powder, made from the dried root. Used to treat both diarrhea and constipation, depending upon the amount given. Purgative, astringent, stomachic, tonic.

• **Sage** *(Salvia officinalis)* - Wound treatment, skin erruptions, headaches, occasionally as sore throat treatment in form of syrup or lozenges ; commonly used in sausage blends.

• **Sassafras** *(Sassafras albidum)* - Root bark tea is a tradtional "blood purifer:" also folk remedy for stomach problems, gout, high blood pressure; wound wash; oil of sassafras used for cough drops, candy flavoring and beverages.

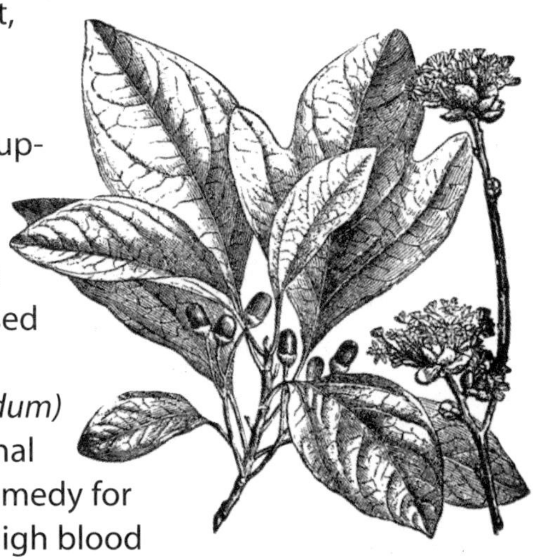

Sassafras
(Sassafras albidum)

• **Saw Palmetto** *(Serenoa repens)* - Historically used in treatment of prostate inflammations, head colds, migraines.

• **Savory** *(Satureja hortensis)* - Used as a wound wash, due to its antibacterial action (learned later in the century); also used similarly to thyme.

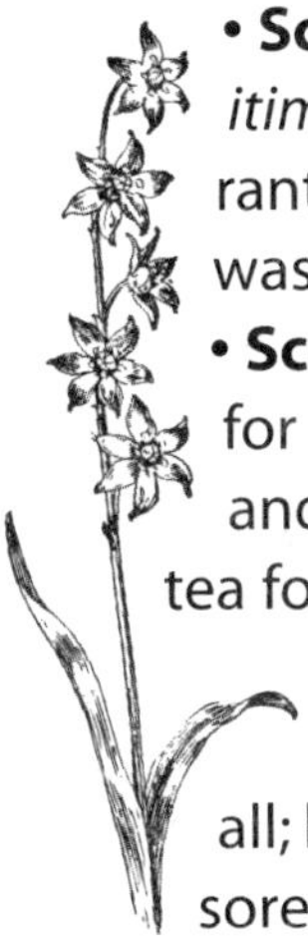

Scilla

• **Scilla** *(Scilla maritima,* some sources list *Urginea maritima)* - Also listed as squill; cardiac stimulant, expectorant in treating croup, colds. As with digitalis, this plant was dangerous if misused or self-administered.

• **Scouring Rush** *(Equisetum hymale & E. arvense)* - Used for scouring pots and pans, removing rust from guns and sabres. Historically used to treat kidney problems, tea for lung lesions from tuberculosis, bladder ailments, urinary problems.

• **Self-heal** *(Prunella vulgaris)* - Often called Heal-all; leaf tea was used as gargle for sore throat, mouth sores, fevers, diarrhea; externally for wounds and ulcers.

• **Sheep Sorrel** *(Rumex acetosella)* - Fevers, inflammation, scurvy, diuretic,

• **Shepherd's Purse** *(Capsella bursa-pastoris)* - Both dried and fresh herb used to stop bleeding and as diuretic and styptic. Tea used for diarrhea and dysentery and externally as wound wash.

• **Skullcap, Mad-dog** *(Scutellaria lateriflora)* - Known as Mad-dog skullcap because the tea was used as remedy for rabies. Decoction or tea was sedative and antispasmodic and used in treating various nervous conditions including sleeplessness, anxiety and epilepsy.

• **Slippery Elm** *(Ulmus rubra)* - Inner bark of indigenous tree, used for relief of coughs, sore throat, laryngitis. Still available for that purpose today in tablet form.

• **Snakeroot, Seneca** *(Polygala senega)* - Root tea used as emetic, expectorant, diuretic, antispasmodic, sweat inducer.

• **Snakeroot, White** *(Eupatorium rugosum)* - Treatment (tea) for ague, diarrhea, painful urination, poultice for snakebite. Very poisonous; causes "milk sickness" which can be fatal if a person drinks milk from cows that have grazed on the plant. Abraham Lincoln's mother is said to have died of milk sickness from drinking milk from a cow that had grazed on white snakeroot.

• **Solomon's Seal** *(Polygonatum biflorum)* - Folk remedy for indigestion lung ailments, debility; roots poulticed for wounds, bruises, sores. Also traditional remedy for piles rheumatism, skin problems, arthritis.

• **Spearmint** *(Mentha spicata)* - Used as treatment for upset stomach, dysentery, diarrhea and as appetite stimulant in debilitating illnesses. Also as flavoring and tea.

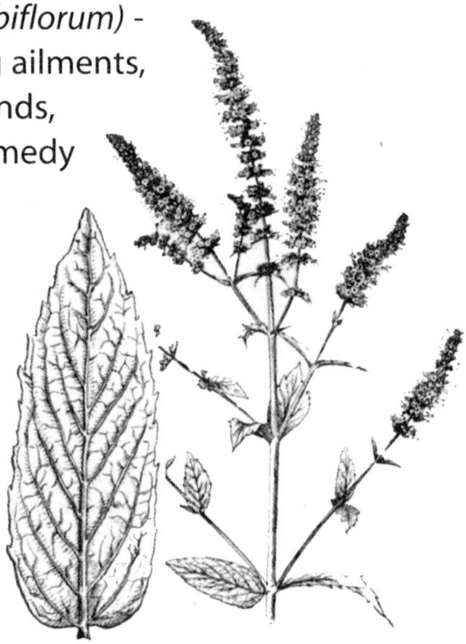

Spearmint *(Mentha spicata)*

• **Spice Bush** *(Lindera benzoin)* - A shrub growing about the size of a lilac bush, in full shade and moist soil; also known as Benjamin bush, feverbush and wild allspice; historically used in treatment for fever and flu. Berries dried and pulverized for allspice substitute in cooking.

• **Spigelia, Pinkroot** *(Spigelia marilandica)* - American Indians as well as physicians, used root tea for expulsion of worms, especially in children and continued in use well into the middle of the 20th century. *See also page 22.*

• **Squaw-Weed** *(Senecio aureus)* - Golden ragwort; Root tea used by American Indians, settlers and physicians to treat chilbirth complications, lung ailments, dysentery, urination difficulties and in treating wounds. Leaves, seed and juice of plant all used.

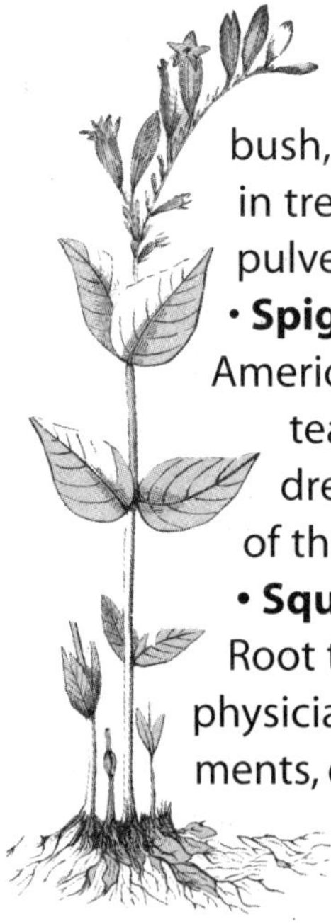

Pinkroot
(Spigelia marilandica)

• **Stinging Nettle** *(Utica dioica)* - Traditionally leaf tea used as blood purifer; diuretic, astringent, for anemia, gout glandular diseases. In older herbals listed as *Jatropha stimulosa;* sometimes used as counter-irritant for rheumatism, arthritis.

• **St. Johnswort** *(Hypericum perforatum)* - Used as sedative, anti-inflammatory; flowers used in tea and tincture as well as in olive oil for wounds, external ulcers.

• **Sumac** *(Rhus glabra, R. typhina)* - Porcher says, *"If the bark of the root is boiled in equal parts of mik and water...it will cure burns without leaving a scar."* Berries also used to make a cooling beverage; substitute (bark) for tannin in tanning hides. An infusion of the leaves, sweetened with honey used as gargle, as well as infusion of the inner bark of the root being employed as a gargle for sore throat. Leaves were used to stop dysentery; root tea was emetic, diuretic. Bark tea formerly used for diarrhea, dysentery, fevers, mouth or throat ulcers; astringent, tonic, antiseptic. (Note: this is different from poison sumac, which has white fruits and grows near swamps).

• **Sunflower** *(Helianths annuus)* - American Indians used tea from the flowers for lung problems; leaf tea given for high fevers; leaves poulticed on snakebite and spider bite. Seeds for food, as well as source for oil.

• **Sweet Birch** *(Betula lenta)* - Like wintergreen, sweet birch contains methyl salicylate and was used as infusion, from bark or leaves, for rheumatism, gout, bladder infecton, anti-inflammatory, analgesic. Oil applied as counterirritant. Source of flavoring for birch beer, a popular regional beverage. Other birches used similarly.

• **Sweet Cicely** *(Osmorhiza longistylis)* - Traditional treatment by American Indians for general debility, tonic for upset stomach, root poulticed on boils and wounds; root tea an eye wash. Also for coughs, stomachaches. Pleasant flavored leaves used in desserts and drinks, as well

• **Swamp Rose-Mallow** *(Hibiscus moscheutos)* - Used as demulcent and emollient in dysentery and urinary and lung ailments.

• **Sweet Gum** *(Liquidambar styraciflua)* - Listed in older medicinal sources as Liquidambar, this is the native sweet gum tree. Resin was used for treating scabies, sometimes used in resolving tumors of the uterus. American Indians used it as wound herb and as a febrifuge. Also a dye herb for coloring cloth gray, for Confederate uniforms.

• **Tansy** *(Tanacetum vulgare)* - As a wound wash for tumors, inflammations, swelling; leaf tea for dyspepsia, flatulence, for expelling worms. Leaves used for insect repellant, especially in deterring ants.

• **Tea, New Jersey** *(Ceanothus americanus)* - Also know as Red Root in old texts. Leaf tea was historically a popular beverage, as well as being used as a sedative and expectorant. Root tea used for dysentery, sore throats, whooping cough, bronchitis.

See also New Jersey Tea, page 20.

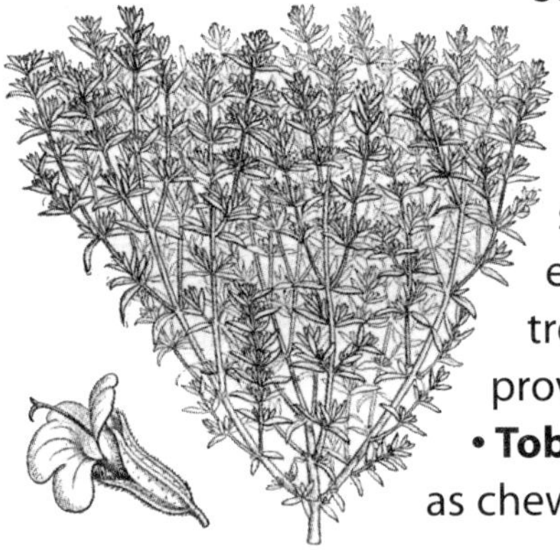

Thyme
(Thymus pulegioides))

• **Thyme** *(Thymus pulegioides)* - Historically used for treating nervous disorders, flu, coughs, stomachaches, as a blood purifier, expectorant, antiseptic and for treating toothaches. Has been proven to have antiseptic properties.

• **Tobacco** *(Nicotiana tabacum)* - Used as chewing and smoking tobacco, this plant also was used for a variety of medicinal purposes. Chewed leaves were applied to insect stings; poultices used for swellings and injuries; used as insecticide on poultry and garden plants.

• **Tomato** *(Solanum lycopersicum)* - Porcher, in 1863, said," The fruit of this plant is well known as an article of food....the use of the fruit tends to promote constipation and prevent diarrhea." Thomas Jefferson is credited with developing the Brandywine tomato variety in the early 1800s.

• **Toothwort** *(Dentaria diphylla)* - Also called toothache root; root peppery, used as folk remedy for toothache, colds, headaches; root tea gargled for sore throats.

• **Upland Evans Root** *(Heuchera americana)*- Usually listed as Alum Root, Crane's Bill or Heuchera; astringent, "destroys canker and humours and stops intestinal fevers..." from ***The Indian Physician***, 1828. Used as wound herb and blood stopping in small wounds. *See also Alumroot, page 10.*

• **Valerian** *(Valeriana officinalis)* - Used to treat depression, insomnia, nervous headaches.

• **Vernonica** *(Veronica officinalis)* - Also listed as Common Speedwell; root or leaf tea used to encourage urination, also in treatment of menstruation, as a blood purifer, for skin and kidney problems, gout, rheumatism. *Veronica gluca*, or Ironweed, used also as blood tonic by American Indians and to regulate menses.

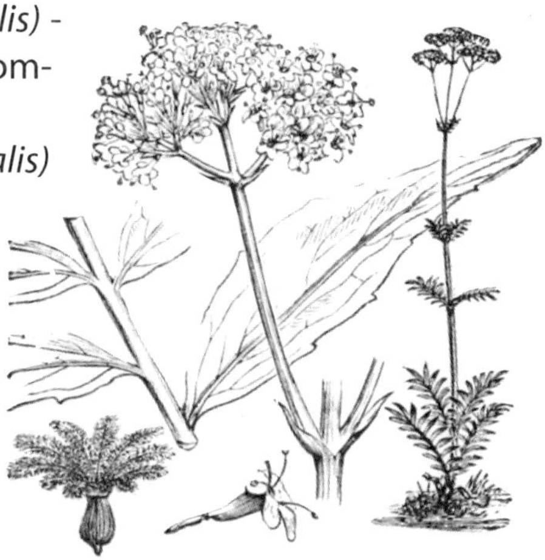
Valerian *(Valeriana officinalis)*

• **Vervain, Blue** *(Verbena hastata)* - Used as women's tonic, as well as for coughs, dysentery, stomach cramps, fevers. Described in ***The Cherokee Physician*** as an emetic, but of less use than some other emetics. Decoction used for treating fevers.

• **Viburnum** *(Virburnum prunifolium)* - Known as Blackhaw; diuretic, uterine tonic, sedative. *V. opulus*, or highbush cranberry, used similarly, as was Possumhaw *(V. nudum)*.

• **Violet** *(Viola tricolor)* - Also called Heartsease and Johnny Jump-Up; Fomerly considered valuable in treating epilepsy, ulcers. Related species, *Viola palmata*, or hand-leaved violet, according to Porcher, was *"employed by negroes for making* *soup and is commonly called wild okra."* The bruised leaves were used as emollient (soothing) to the skin, to reduce abraisions. Traditionally in folk medicine considered diuretic, blood purifer, used for asthma, skin erruptions, eczema.

• **Wahoo** *(Euonymous atropupureus & E. americanus)* - Root tea used for vomiting of blood, painful urination, wash for swollen limbs; bark used as tonic, laxative, expectorant; used briefly for malaria, as well as indigestion, constipation. powdered bark applied to scalp for dandruff. Fruit, seeds and bark considered poisonous.

• **Walnut, Black** *(Juglans nigra)* - Lint dripped in oil from kernal and applied to toothache; tea, of leaves, used for scrofulous conditions.

• **Willow** *(Salix nigra, S. alba)* - Pain reliever, headaches; substitute for quinine in emergencies although not effective for that purpose; purgative and vermifuge.

• **Wintergreen** *(Gaultheria procumbens)* - Used like aspirin and willow bark, for pain reliever. Contains methyl salicylate.

• **Witch-Hazel** *(Hamamelis virginiana)* - Teas used for colds, sore throats; twig tea used as wash to keep muscles limber; tea also used for dysentery, coughing; used externally for bruises, muscle soreness; distilled and used for eyewash, ointments, skin refresher. Source of material for healing salve.

• **Wood Betony** *(Pedicularis canadensis)* - Also known as Lousewort; root tea used for stomachache and diarrhea; used in cough medicines, poultices for tumors, sore muscles, swellings.

• **Wood Sage** *(Teucrium canadense)* - Also known as Germander and Wild Basil. Used for lung ailments, worms, piles; as wound herb and gargle as well as to induce urination and sweating.

• **Wormwood** *(Artemisia absinthium)* - Tea used for fevers, as worm expellent, gall bladder and liver ailments, leaves nibbled to stimulate appetite.

• **Yam, Wild** *(Dioscorea villosa)* - Dried root tea used to relieve labor pains in women. Fresh root tea used for colic, asthma, rheumatism.

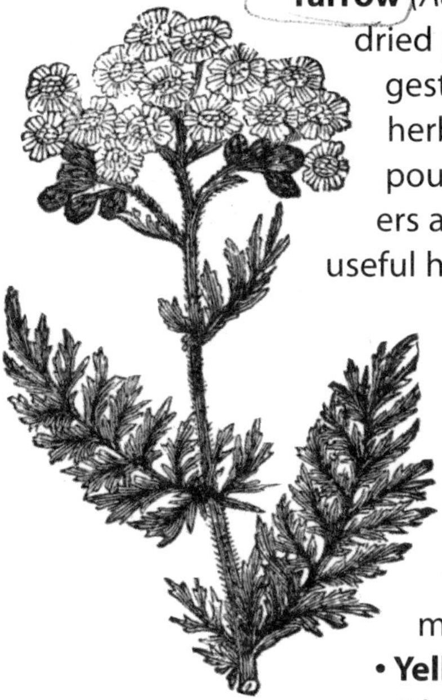

Yarrow
(Achillea millefolium)

• **Yarrow** *(Achillea millefolium)* - Tea from dried plant, used for fevers, colds, indigestion, stomach problems. Fresh herb used as a blood stopping poultice, also dried, powdered flowers and leaves used as styptic. Very useful herb for stopping bleeding. Use as battlefield wound herb dates from early Greek and Roman times. Named for Achilles, who died of a wound to the heel and who supposedly bled to death. This plant was an important medicine to folk healers for millenia.

• **Yellow Giant Hyssop** *(Agastache nepetoides)* - Traditional treatment for poison ivy rash.

• **Yellow Root** *(Hydrastis canadensis)* - Golden seal; also known by names of Yellow Puccoon, Indian Paint, Eye Balm, Yellow Eye and Jaundice Root. Was listed as early as 1798 in medical pharmacopeas, although Native Americans had been using it for centuries. See Goldenseal, listed earlier in this plant text. Note: another plant, also called Yellowroot *(Xanthorhiza simplicissima)* is used as an astringent, antimicrobial, etc. but is a different plant.

• **Yellow Adder's-tongue** *(Erythronium americanum)* - Also known as Trout-Lily, Dog-Tooth Violet; Root poulticed to reduce swelling; large doses are emetic. Pharmaceopea as late as 1927 listed Yellow Adder's-Tongue as "used like colchicum" in treating gout.

Specific Mixtures and Terms Found in Civil War Physicians's References

• **Anodynes** - Remedies against pain.

• **Antimony** - *"A brittle, whitish metal, usually found associated with sulphur. This supposedly comes from anti-moine, derived from the fatal effects upon some monks upon whom its properties were tried by Valentine,"* ***Dictionary of Terms Used in Medicine,*** 1846.

• **Antimonial Powder** - *"This pharmacopoeial preparation is an oxdide of antimony combined with phosphate of lime. It is used as a substitute for James' Powder,"* ***Dictionary of Medical Terms,*** 1846. Used as purgative and for fevers.

• **Birdlime** - From the inner bark of *Ilex aquifolium*, of Europe; used as an emetic.

• **Blue Mass** - A mixture of mercury, calomel (mercurous chloride) strychnine, opium and acetate of lead, used to treat diarrhea and dysentery. Commonly used by physicians during the Civil War period, but lethal and did more harm than good.

• **Cathartic** - A cathartic agent, especially a laxative.

• **Diseremus Pills** - Equal amounts of resin and red pepper for diarhea. First concocted by an Alabama medical officer.

• **Diuretic** - Any drug or plant used to induce the passing of urine.

• **Dover's Compound** - A powdered drug, made of ipecac and opium, formerly used to relive pain and induce perspiration; named for Thomas Dover, 1660-1742.

• **Emetic** - A substance which causes vomiting.

• **Emmenagogue** - A medicine that induces the menstrural flow.

• **Emollient** - Softening and smoothing to the skin.

• **Faynard's Powder** - A celebrated powder for stopping hemorrhage, said to have been nothing more than the charcoal of beech wood, finely powdered.

• **Flux** - To cause to flow

• **Gregory's Powde**r - Contains rhubarb, light magnesia and ginger; used for treating intestinal problems.

• **Humour** - In medieval physiology, one of the four fluids of the body: blood, phlegm, choler, and black bile, the dominance of which was thought to determine a person's character and good health.

• **Intermittent Fever** - Malaria; also known historically as marsh fever in Europe and jungle fever in India. *"The malaris of Campagna is the name of an endemic intermittent, arising from the aria cattiva, as it is called, exhaled from decaying vegetables in the neighbourhood of Rome, especially about the marshes."* Remember, until after the Civil War, it wasn't known that mosquitoes carried malaria;"miasmas" from the swamps and poor diet were all believed to be sources of malaria.

• **James' Powder** - A celebrated fever powder, supposed to be similiar to the Antimonii oxidum cum phosphate calcis, or antimonial powder.

• **Mercurial Pills** - *"Pilulae hydrargyri or blue pill; a mass consisting of mercury rubbed with confection of red roses until the globules can no longer be seen, and then blended with liquorice* (sic) *powder."* ***Dictionary of Medical Terms,*** 1846.

• **Moxa** - *"A small mass of combustible vegetable matter, prepared from the* Artemisia moxa, *or Moxa-weed, a Chinese plant of the order Compsitæ, and employed as an actual cautery. European moxa, usually made with cotton-wool which has been soaked in a solution of nitrate of chlorate of potash; or the pith of the* Helianthus annus, *or sunflower, which contains naturally nitrate of potash."* ***Dictionary of Terms Used in Medicine,*** 1846.

• **Mustard Plaster** - Black mustard seed which was ground, mixed with water to wash away some of the oils, dried, then applied in cloth or paper, directly to moistened skin where it produced a warming sensation in five minutes. Generally used for sprains, injured muscles, arthritis, etc.

• **Nervine** - That which relieves disorders of the nerves, such as antispasmodics and others.

• **Oak-Apple** - Gall of the oak tree; used in making ink; often the doctor was responsible for the keeping formulas such as this.

• **Officinal** - *"A term applied to any medicines directed by the colleges to be kept in the shops."* ***Dictionary of Terms Used in Medicine,*** 1846. Plants which contain the name, officianle, as part of the botanical name (such as *Hyssopus officinalis*, traditionally used as gargle for sore throat, tea to relive gas, stomaches, used with horehound for bronchitis and coughs), designates it as the official plant hyssop that was used and recognized medicinally.

• **Onion** - According to Sylvia Windle Humphrey, in ***A Matter of Taste,*** The Macmillan Co., 1965, p. 161, onions were so important that in 1864 General Ulysses S. Grant said, *"I will not move my army without onions."* Onions were seen as such an important battlefield wound medicine as well as useful in intestinal problems that he refused to move his soldiers into battle without a supply. Two days later he reportedly received three train car loads of onions.

In *Letter from a Country Girl,* by Jackson, a widely reprinted story in the Civil War, which prompted posters, girls were advised, *"Don't send your sweetheart a love letter, send him an onion."*

• **Opodeldoc** - A solution of soap in alcohol, with the addition of camphor and volataile oils.

• **Paragoric** - Tincture of opium, used for pain killer.

• **Pearl Eye** - Pearl in the eye, the old English name for cataract.

• **Permanent Ink** - Doctors, especially military physicians, often kept formulas for things like dyes for making military uniforms the right color, shoe polish and inks. Permanent ink was a solution of nitrate of silver, thickened with sap green or cochineal. Common ink was made by adding an infusion or decoction of the nut gall to sulphate of iron, dissolved in water. Red ink was composed of Brazil wood, gum and alum. Printers ink was a black paint made of linseed or nut oil and lamp black.

• **Purgative** - Any material given to promote evacuation of the bowels.

• **Rubefacient** - A substance that irriates the skin, causing redness. Hot pepper oil, an ingredient in over the counter arthritis and sore muscle creams, is an example.

• **Seneca Oil** - Petroleum oil that bubbles to the surface on springs in New York and Ohio, which was bottled and sold as a topical medicine for skin ailments and disorders.

• **Stag Horn** - Used medicinally for lack of sexual appetite; the horn was generally burned to an ash and that was given in brandy or whiskey.

• **Vermifuge** - An agent that destroys or removes intestinal worms.

• **Vulnerary** - Used in the healing or treating of wounds.

• **Web** - Spider's webs were sometimes collected for use as wound dressing when bandages could not be found.

Bibliography

A Dictionary of Terms Used in Medicine, Isaac Hays, M.D., 1855.
A Dictionary of Terms Used in Medicine, Isaac Hays, M.D., 1846.
Civil War Plants & Herbs, Patricia B. Mitchell, 1996.
Collections for an Essay Towards a Materia Medica of the United States, Benjamin Smith Barton, 1798.
Commerce on the Prairies, Josiah Gregg, 1844.
Dates of Selected Inventions and Occurrences, Virginia Mescher, Nature's Finest, Burke, VA, 1998.
Did They Eat That? Virginia Mescher, 1999.
Herbal Medicines on the Santa Fe Trail, Jim Long, Long Creek Herbs, 1996.
Hoblyn's Medical Dictionary, Issac Hays, M.C., 1855.
"It will do no harm to try it," the Diary of Elias Slagle, 1859, edited by Jim Long.
Inventions & Occurrences During the Latter Part of the 18th Century, Virginia Mescher, 1994.
Materia Medica and Pharmacology, David M.R. Culbreth, PhG., MD., 1927.
Peterson Field Guide to Medicinal Plants, Steven Foster & James A. Duke, 1990.
Resources of the Southern Fields and Forests, a Medical Botany of the Confederate States, Francis P. Porcher, 1863, Steam-Power Press of Evans & Cogswell, Charleston; Reprinted by Arno & The New York Times, 1970.
Squires Companion to the British Pharmacopea, 1894.
The Big Book of Herbs, Arthur O. Tucker, Ph.D. and Thomas Debaggio, Interweave Press, 2000.
The Expansion of Everyday Life, 1860-1876; Daniel E. Sutherland, Harper & Row. 1990.
The Indian Physician, Jonas Rishel, 1828; Reprinted 1987 by Friends of the Libraries of The Ohio State University.
Young's Great Book of Secrets, 1872, F. E. Phelan.

Index